SOTHIS PRESS

Sothis Press aims to completely reimagine the public domain book with an emphasis on universal access to captivatingly designed print editions. We believe that technology will enable every single book ever published to be perpetually accessible in beautiful print form. Sothis is beauty in ubiquity.

www.sothis.press
1 Waterhouse Square, London, ECIN 2ST

Brunker's Carminative Balsam

Globe Medicine Company

SOTHIS PRESS

ISBN 978-1-83548-892-8

This edition is published by
Sothis Press © 2023. The company
is registered in England and Wales.
The Company Number is 14900389.

BRUNKER'S Carminative BALSAM

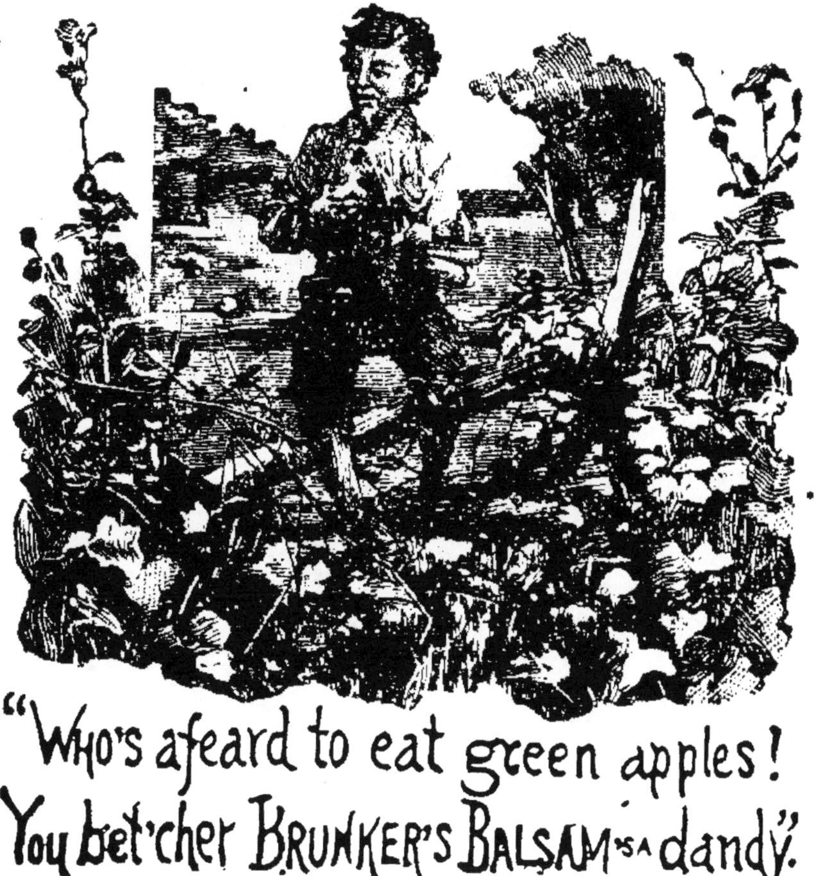

"Who's afeard to eat green apples! You bet'cher BRUNKER'S BALSAM's a dandy".

[LETTER FROM DR. BRUNKER.]

Having disposed of my entire interest in Brunker's Carminative Balsam to the Globe Medicine Co., of Terre Haute, Ind., all orders should hereafter be addressed to them.

The character of the gentlemen composing the Company is a sufficient guarantee that the high standard attained by Brunker's Carminative Balsam will be faithfully maintained.

The public can rest assured that the formula will be rigidly adhered to in every particular, and the efficiency of the Balsam remain unimpaired by the change in ownership.

Thanking you for the confidence and patronage extended to me in the past, and soliciting for my sucessors the same kindly consideration, with the most sincere wishes for your success and happiness, I remain sincerely your friend,

50,000

DIE EVERY YEAR!

FIFTY THOUSAND DIE annually in this country from disorders of the stomach and bowels alone. Three-fourths of this vast number are children under five years of age, many of whom might, no doubt, be saved by the timely use of proper remedies.

WHAT TO DO, is a question that is not easily solved. It has been asked thousands of times by many a despairing heart, as it has hopelessly watched some loved one fading day by day into death without the ability to do anything to stay the destroyer's hand.

WHAT HAS BEEN DONE has too often proven itself an actual

harm instead of a benefit. The kindly processes of nature have been disregarded and subverted; her beseeching cry for bread has been answered with a stone; what she asked and needed to repair the waste has been cruelly withheld, under the mistaken idea that human wisdom was above hers.

INSTEAD OF AIDING NATURE to throw off the offending causes, the efforts of the physician and of many "patent nostrums," has been directed too often to damming up the source of the trouble within the system by the use of astringents, and there permitting it to fester and destroy the life of the sufferer.

A THOROUGH UNDERSTANDING of the nature and cause of any disease is necessary before it is possible to intelligently treat it. Anything short of this is blind empiricism, and consequently unworthy of confidence. Let us, therefore, inquire into these matters, that we may be prepared to determine what should be done—and how.

EVERY CASE of Flux, Summer Complaint, Diarrhœa, Cramp Colic,

Cholera Morbus, &c., is due, either directly or indirectly, to the presence and *fermentation* of indigestible and irritating substances in the stomach and bowels, or to external irritating causes, such as colds, teething, etc., resulting, in either case, in congestion, inflammation and unnatural action, and, if not controlled, in suppuration of the parts involved.

UNDER SUCH conditions it would be clearly wrong to undertake, by the use of astringents, to arrest the discharge and allow the cause to remain. It would also be equally foolish, though less harmful, to pour into the already irritated and distressed stomach and bowels fiery draughts of some vile compound under the mistaken idea that "the stomach needs warming." It invariably aggravates the trouble.

THE PROPER COURSE to pursue is to neutralize the acid in the stomach and bowels, soothe and quiet the pain and irritation, and by a gentle, kindly action of the bowels, remove the cause of the trouble, and the case is practically cured. Such are the properties and invariable action of

BRUNKER'S

CARMINATIVE BALSAM

We Guarantee Every Bottle to Give Satisfaction,

And do just what we claim for it in Summer Complalut, Diarrhœa, Cramp Colic, Flux, Cholera Morbus, Congestion, and Neuralgia of the Stomach and Bowels.

PRICE, 25 AND 50 CENTS.

(*Holding two to five ounces respectively.*)

SOLD BY DRUGGISTS AND DEALERS GENERALLY.

If your druggist or dealer does not keep it, they can procure it from almost any wholesale druggist or from us direct.

The Small Size will be sent by mail on receipt of price and six cents to pay postage.

MANUFACTURED ONLY BY THE

GLOBE MEDICINE CO.

Terre Haute, Ind.

DIRECTIONS:

DOSE FOR ADULT.—One to two table-spoonfuls.

DOSE FOR CHILDREN.—10 to 14 years of age, half to a tablespoonful.

DOSE FOR CHILDREN.—5 to 10 years of age, two to three teaspoonfuls.

DOSE FOR INFANTS.—Half teasponful or more.

No danger in taking an overdose. Don't drink any water immediately after taking the medicine. For infants and children it may be given in a little sweetened water.

IN SUMMER COMPLAINT—The dose should be repeated every hour or two. Keep the bowels warm by covering them with a flannel bandage. Keep the child in a cool room, and when possible, in the open air. Continne the Balsam until fully rocovered.

IN DIARRHŒA—In mild cases take full doses, repeated every two hours. In severe cases take large doses, repeated every half hour until controlled, and then lessen the dose and lengthen the intervals, until well. The patient should remain as quiet as possible.

IN DYSENTERY or FLUX—Take full doses every half hour or hour, until the griping and bearing down pain is relieved, then smaller doses at longer intervals until well. Keep off the feet, remain quiet, keep the bowels warm, and avoid too much water.

IN CRAMP COLIC—Take large doses, and in severe cases repeat every half hour until relieved. Keep quiet, and if the bowels do not move in five or six hours after the use of the Balsam, take a dose of castor oil with a teaspoonful of paregoric in it.

IN CHOLERA MORBUS—Take the larger dose named for the age and repeat every half hour until relieved. If the patient is very weak give small doses of brandy or whisky every hour for a while, then substitute quinine in place of the stimulants every three hours. Continue the use of the Balsam at intervals until fully recovered.

IN CONGESTION and NEURALGIA of the Stomach and Bowels take large doses every hour or oftener. Keep the parts warm by the application of warm fomentations, or hot flannel cloths. Use hot applications to the feet. When the paroxysm is relieved give three-grain doses of quinine every two hours for six or eight hours.

IN INDIGESTION, with sour stomach and belching, nothing can act with better effect. Take about half a tablespoonful immediately before each meal. Season the food well with salt. Avoid eating anything that causes distress—a milk diet is usually the best.

FOR THE BABIES.

BRUNKER'S CARMINATIVE BALsam being composed of soothing and healing spices and gums, combined with antacids, is perfectly harmless to the most delicate infant. We guarantee that no harm will result from the largest possible overdose, as it contains no narcotic or astringent properties.

DR BRUNKER, after thirty years' experience in the use of the Balsam in thousands of cases, says of it: "This medicine should be in every nursery in the land, and I guarantee that the benefits resulting from one year's use of the Balsam will secure from any mother a testimonial of unqualified endorsement, beyond anything that I have ever claimed for it."

IF THE CHILD IS FRETFUL, colicky, teething, the milk curdles in its stomach, has unnatural or offensive passages from the bowels, the urine scalds or chafes the private parts, the abdomen hot or swollen, breath offensive, give half a teaspoonful of Brunker's Balsam in a little sweetened water, every two or three hours, and you will be surprised at the result.

DON'T conclude that the dear little sufferer "has worms" every time it shows some of the symptoms given above. Worm medicine destroys more children than it saves, and should never be given except under the direction of a physician. NEVER give worm medicines during the months that diarrhœa is prevalent.

TESTIMONIALS.

We could give thousands of testimonials if our space would permit and it was necessary, but we feel that the best evidence in the world as to the character of an individual is what his neighbors say of him, and so it is with a medicine. Below we print a few expressions from some of the leading druggists of Terre Haute, Ind., and from persons who have used Brunker's Balsam themselves or in their families. The character and standing of these persons can not be questioned. Any of them will cheerfully answer any inquiries concerning the merits of the medicines.

I have sold Brunker's Balsam for the past fifteen years, and can truthfully say that it has proven the most efficacious and the best selling remedy that I ever sold. JAS. E. SOMES,
Druggist, Cor. Sixth and Ohio Sts.

Brunker's Balsam is one of the staple family medicines with our trade. Its sale has been attended with satisfaction to both buyer and seller.

BUNTIN DRUG CO., ,
Cor. Main and Sixth Sts.

We have always found Brunker's Balsam a good seller, and to give good satisfaction. OAK HALL PHARMACY,
Cor. Seventh and Main Sts.

Our house has sold Brunker's Balsam during the past sixteen years. The sales have steadily increased, and to-day we regard it as standard. We have no hesitancy in recommending it. GULICK & CO.,
Druggists, Cor. Fourth and Main Sts.

Brunker's Balsam outsells any preparation of its kind I have ever handled. D. P. COX,
Druggist, Cor. Eighth and Main Sts.

Our sales on Brunker's Carminative Balsam have, for several years, exceeded the combined sales of all other preparations of its class, and has given complete satisfaction to our trade.

E. H. BINDLEY & CO.,
Wholesale Druggist, 666 Main St.

Brunker's Balsam gives general satisfaction. Purchasers always speak in

the highest terms of its merits. It outsells all other preparations of its class with me. JOS. S. MADISON,
Druggist, Cor. Third and Park Sts.

Brunker's Balsam is undoubtedly a happy combination for correcting the ailments for which it is recommended. For many years it has proven a safe and efficient remedy.

J. & C. BAUR,
Druggists, Cor. Wabash Ave and 7th.

We have sold Brunker's Balsam for the past twenty years, and fail to recall a single instance in that time wherein it has failed to give entire satisfaction. We believe its record is without a parallel.

COOK, BELL & LOWRY,
Wholesale Druggists, 611 and 613 Main St. New York Office, 32 Platt St.

Brunker's Balsam is the only thing I have ever found to give relief in nervous dyspepsia. We are never without it in our family, and regard it as a panacea for the ailments peculiar to childhood. JAS. A. SCUDDER,
Trav. Salesman Joe Strong's Coffee and Spice Mills.

I regard **Brunker's Balsam** as the most effectual preparation in all the derangements for which it is recommended. My wife and I believe that it saved the life of our little child after all other means tried had failed to accomplish any good. We would not be without it. C. C. LUCKY,
Trav. Salesman Bement, Rea & Co.,
Wholesale Grocers.

When in the drug trade I sold Brunker's Balsam, and recommended it on its merits, and never had a case where it failed to give satisfaction. I have used it in my family for the last seven years, and regard it as the *best* remedy in the market for the diseases for which it is intended, either in children or adults. Yours truly,
WILL W. ADAMSON,
Dealer in Window Glass and Painters' Supplies, South Sixth St.

Have used Brunker's Balsam in my family for cholera morbus and like complaints. It acts like a charm; would not be without it in the house.
HENRY J. VOGES,
Prop'r Barber Shop, 653 Wabash Ave.

I sell stacks of Brunker's Balsam. Sold at least two gross last year. I re gard it as a very excellent preparation, especially so for children.

CAPT. J. H. ALLEN,
Druggist, 500 North Thirteenth St.

We have sold Brunker's Balsam for years, and never knew of any preparation that gave such general satisfaction. Never had a complaint from any one, and sells ahead of all other similar preparations combined.

W. D. WAGGONER,
Druggist, 1201 East Main St.

My sales on Brunker's Balsam are good. It gives perfect satisfaction as far as I am aware; never had a complaint. Parties who once use it invariably call for it again.

ALBERT NEUKOM,
Druggist, 1241 Wabash Ave.

We have used Brunker's Balsam in our own family, and Mrs. Johnson and myself have recommended it to hundreds of others, and never knew it to fail in a single instance. We believe that it saved the life of our little child in a severe case of summer complaint, after we had nearly abandoned all hope of its recovery. We are never without a bottle of it in the house, and I always keep some in the locker of the baggage car on any train. Have often given it to passengers who have been suddenly seized with cholera morbus and like complaints, and always with the happiest results. It is certainly a wonderful remedy.

WASH. JONHSON,
Conductor T. H. & I. Railroad.

Having used Brunker's Carminative Balsam for our children for summer complaint and stomach troubles, we heartily endorse it, and recommend it to all parents who have children thus afflicted. We would not be without it. Yours respectfully,

MR. AND MRS. J. A. FRYBURGER,
108 South Fourth St.

Have been troubled for several years with attacks of cramps and congestion of the stomach. Never found anything to give me relief until I tried Brunker's Balsam, which gives me almost instant relief. I have recommended it to many others for similar troubles, including summer complaint and diarrhœa, and never knew of it to fail in a single instance.

JOHN W. FUNK,
Proprietor of Barber Shop, 1111 East Main St.

Hollingsworth's A. & S. (Alterant and Solvent) solves acid accretions in the blood, alters the thickened and diseased membrane, removes all impurities from the blood, invigorates the general system, gives tone to the liver, kidneys and bowels, removes all disease germs from the system, clears and beautifies the skin and enriches the blood. Price, $1.00.

Hollingsworth's Demulcent keeps the nostrils cool and open, prevents the formation of dry crusts, scales and scabs, allays inflammation and heals the membrane. Price, 50c.

Hollingsworth's Antipyretic promptly stops a FRESH COLD, a paroxysm of sneezing, asthma or tickling cough. We guarantee that it will stop a fresh cold in twenty minutes, and completely break it up within twenty-four hours; that it will stop a paroxysm of sneezing, asthma or tickling cough in ten minutes. *We mean just what we say.* Price, 75c.

SOLD VERY GENERALLY BY DRUGGISTS.

Spotted something that isn't quite right?

Let us know and we'll fix it for future reprints. And as a thank you for your diligence, we'll send you a free Sothis book of your choice.

publisher@sothis.press

This page intentionally left blank

Made in United States
Orlando, FL
04 November 2026

90201489R00016